A Book of Elliptical Workouts

Discover How to Exercise Your Entire Body and Never Get Bored on Your Elliptical Machine

by Lukas Taylor

Table of Contents

Introduction

Most people that work out on an elliptical machine simply hop on and get moving, perhaps occasionally adjusting the resistance and incline settings. But did you know that there are countless other *specific exercise routines* that you can do on an elliptical machine that will give you so much variety that you'll never get bored? Not only that, but you can target specific parts of your body with certain workouts, enough so that you can actually exercise your entire body on just this one machine.

This book will provide you with detailed instructions for 9 exercise routine variations that you can do on the elliptical so that you can choose what to do each day depending on your mood or your workout objective. The exercise routines are described using a 30 minute session time-frame which, if done daily, is going to noticeably burn fat and tone muscle. If you're one to prefer longer workouts, then you can simply stretch out the time frame, or double up workouts per session. If you're ready to learn how to make the most out of your elliptical machine, let's get started!

Part 1: FAT BURNING

Chapter 1: The Beginner Workout

This is the workout to do when you are just starting out. It's a very simple workout, but it is also intense, and works out all your muscle groups. Before you jump in, it is important that you are properly prepared. Loose-fitting clothes are ideal, but if you want to wear tight-fitting clothes, then it is best to wear clothes that can breathe. Ensure that you are hydrated as well, and wear shoes that have comfortable soles. Even though your feet will be anchored to the platforms, having enough padding will ensure that your feet don't get tired before you do.

Pre-Workout

Now it's time to step on to the machine. You will see two platforms to place your feet, two handles that move along with your feet, and a set of handles that remain in a stationary position. Hold on to the stationary handles and place one foot on the platform farthest away from you first. So, if you are entering from the left of the machine, put your right foot on the right platform, which would be the one farthest from you. Then, place your left foot on the left platform. Before you make your first step, ensure that the platform that you will step on first is lowered to prevent mishaps or accidents. Steady yourself after getting both feet up before starting the machine. Ensure that your feet are aligned with your hips, and are turned straight forward.

The elliptical is activated by kinetic energy, so you must start pedaling in order for the screen to come on. Ensure that you are standing straight (not hunched over or anything like that) when you are using this machine. The screen should come on, and you will see the options to set your weight, the distance you want to go, the mode you want to use, the time you'll spend, etc. The three most important settings to get right are your weight, the duration of the session and the intensity of the workout. With modes, you can set how your workouts will be structured. The best to do is a random workout, where it alternates between intensities, but for this simple workout, you won't need any incline or up the resistance.

Minute 1

As a first timer, it is best for you to start off at level one and remain there. Set the time for 30 minutes, and start pedaling. You pedal by doing a motion as if you are walking. Your arms and legs will alternate in tandem. It will feel awkward at first and unnatural, but you will get the hang of it. Ensure your legs aren't too locked into position, as you will still need to move around your knees a little. Since this is a simple workout throughout, the only change you will make is your own speed.

Minute 2

Increase your speed to as high as you can and maintain it for the next 3-4 minutes. Make sure it is a speed that you can maintain for that amount of time.

Minute 5

This is where you 'rest', by slowing down to a pace where you can catch your breath. Hold it there for another 5 minutes, and go back to your highest speed by the 10th minute. Keep alternating like this every 5 minutes until the 25th minute.

Minute 25

Slow down to a moderate or slow pace. Keep this pace until the 30th minute or until you are ready to come off of the machine. When you finish, dismount the elliptical the same way that you went on—one foot at a time.

As you grow in sync with the elliptical and find 30-minute workouts don't challenge you anymore, don't up the time length. Instead, you can up the ante by increasing the intensity of the workout. Increasing to higher levels of resistance will force your muscles to work even more to complete the task.

Now that you have learned the basics, it is time to move on and learn more advanced workouts. A lot of these workouts will be achieved by the use of preset modes.

Chapter 2: High Intensity Interval Training

Here you can use preset modes, or do it on your own accord. High-Intensity Interval Training or HIIT is characterized by a short period of very intense workouts, followed by a rest period before repeating the process, hence the name. This method of exercise develops your cardiovascular system and also builds muscle in the process. This sort of cardio burns fat faster than your average cardio workout. Athletes and other very fit people train this way, and it is very effective. Many people do these exercises on the field and the court, but here you will be aided with the elliptical machine.

Pre-Workout

The first step in doing this is to step on to the elliptical the same way you did in the last chapter. With high-intensity interval training, you are doing high intensity stuff, followed by a 'rest' period of low intensity workouts. With the machine, you can speed up and slow down as you like.

Here, I will discuss the Tabata style of HIIT workouts, where you work the machine for a longer time than you rest.

Minute 1

Turn up the resistance level of the machine and pedal at a very fast rate, the fastest rate you can go, and hold it there for 3-4 minutes. Ensure that it is a level that you can only maintain for that amount of time, and no less. Then slow down and pedal at a low rate for about 1 minute. This is the time you're resting, but this kind of rest is different as you won't be stopping. During this time you should be able to catch your breath and prepare for your next intensive round. Ensure that the resistance level setting in your machine is also decreased during your rest time.

Minute 6

Increase the intensity again, and repeat the previous steps. Make sure that you don't completely stop. Decrease the resistance to the lowest levels in your recovery periods if you feel that you are running out of juice. You can also decrease the resistance level in work periods if you feel you won't last for the full 30 minutes.

Minute 25

Do a very light pedal to get your heart rate down for about five minutes or until you are ready to step off of the machine.

Chapter 3: The Hill Climber

Here you will definitely be using the aid of a preset in the machine. With this workout, you will be mimicking a climb up a rocky mountain. Why go to the Himalayas when you can climb Mount Everest in your own home? Choose a preset that increases the resistance and/or the height over a 4-minute period. You are not done after that 4-minute period though, as that is actually where you will be resting.

Pre-Workout

To start, you will need to put your arms either on the stationary handles, or on the middle of the swinging handles. By doing this, you will be hitting your lower back muscles, which will mimic a rowing action.

Minute 1

Start working out at a fast rate for 3 to 4 minutes. Do not depend too much on your legs for this exercise, and make sure you are utilizing your arms and back to control the machine. Then slow down and maintain a slow pace for about a minute.

Minute 6

Repeat the previous step. You will repeat the whole sequence one more time after this step, because things will be shaken up a bit by the 15th minute.

Minute 15

Place your hands at the very top of the handles. In this position, you will be doing a lot of pulling and pushing. As a matter of fact, you will definitely feel the work in your arms in this position. If you are having a difficult time with this, it helps if you lean forward and press down hard on the handles to get your body to push through. Just like before, you will have 3-4 minutes of high intensity work, followed by one minute of cooling off. Be prepared to do this until the 30th minute this time.

Minute 30

Complete a 5-minute cool off before you step off of the machine. To get your cells burning the max amount of calories, ensure that you stay pedaling at a slow rate.

You can also vary the hill climber by pedaling backwards in the second half of the workout. So, in the first half, you will be pedaling forward like you would any other time. Then, in the second half, pedal backwards, like you would be walking backwards on a hill. It will feel weird at first but you will definitely feel the difference in the muscle groups that are being worked out. Here you would have started at the highest intensity then worked down to where you started.

Chapter 4: The Ladder Routine

For this exercise, you will not be splitting evenly between the elliptical machine and your own body weight. This is a full workout in and of itself so if you use this routine in your elliptical just to warm up, keep in mind that it is not recommended unless you know what you are doing. This exercise will work your quads and hamstrings the most, but will give you the all-round fat-burning cardio workout that you need.

Pre-Workout

For this workout, it is best to start off with a 5-minute warm-up. This warm-up should be a simple workout that doesn't involve great resistance or ramp. Do 4 minutes at a moderate pace, and then sprint for the final minute. Most elliptical machines have it programmed to do a cool off for about 2 minutes after a five minute workout. If not, you can do it by yourself.

Minute 1

Now that you have warmed up, it is time to start the actual workout. You will be splitting this workout into three sets. So if you are doing a total of 30 minutes on this workout, you will be allotting 10 minutes for each set. In each of these sets, you will be doing three intervals and they should be divided equally. For the first 3 minutes (in this case, it could be more or less depending on how long you decide your workout should be), you should have a low ramp and a low resistance. Keep a moderately high speed. If you go too fast, you will burn out before too quickly. This workout will take everything out of you.

Minute 4

Here in the second interval, have a medium ramp and medium resistance, and keep a speed that you can maintain for that amount of time.

Minute 7

Here in the third interval, set a high ramp and high resistance. Slow down for a minute after that and, then, get off of the elliptical. Do about 25 squats with your own body weight. Your legs should be burning by now, and if it's not burning, then it should start to do so.

Get back onto the elliptical, but this time, you will be doing it a little different. In the previous steps, you did the squats after you did some sets on the elliptical, but here you will be doing the squats between each interval. Before you get off of the machine after each interval, you must ensure that you slow down for a minute. When you complete the whole sequence, you should barely have any energy left.

Minute 30

Jog at a very slow pace for 2-5 minutes.

Chapter 5: Mile Repeats

For this workout, you will be interacting a lot with your machine's interface. You will be manually increasing and decreasing the intensity and ramp of the machine.

Pre-Workout

Start off by doing a mild warm-up for 5 minutes. You can do it the same way as described in the previous chapter, by doing 4 minutes at a moderate pace, then doing a high pace in the final minute.

Minute 1

After the warm-up, start off your workout by setting the ramp at a low level and a low resistance. Here you will be pedaling at a very fast rate, as fast as you can. You will be doing this for five minutes, so don't put too much into it that you burn out in 3 minutes. Ensure that you devote a minute to cooling off.

Minute 6

After this, step the ramp up to medium, and let the resistance remain the same. However, this time you will be pedaling backward. Do this for 3-4 minutes, and devote some time to cooling off.

Minute 11

After that five minutes is up, increase the ramp to high, and start pedaling forward again. Do this for a good amount of time, and then take a minute to cool off.

After this, you'll start lowering the ramp. Lower the ramp to medium, but keep your speed high and the resistance the same. After five minutes, bring the ramp down to the lowest point, but with medium resistance this time. Here you will be pedaling backwards at a rapid rate. At the end, cool down for 5 minutes.

Part 2: MUSCLE BUILDING

Chapter 6: Strengthening Your Core

One look at the elliptical and immediately you know that it works out your legs and arms. But, did you know that you can get a better core on the elliptical? Yes, sure, burning fat in general will help you get a better looking core, but using the machine in the right way will force the action of your core. Your core is responsible for keeping you upright and balanced, and along with your glutes, are the major muscles responsible for why humans can stand straight compared to other primates.

To get your core worked out, you will have to be in a position that your abs kick in to keep you balanced and upright. To do this, make sure you stretch and you're physically and mentally prepared for the task ahead of it. If you are not a fitness nut, then the next parts will be a bit confusing to you, but try and picture what I am saying.

You will position yourself on the elliptical like you would've before, by keeping your back straight and your feet flat on each platform. This time, you will have to draw your belly button in, raising your chest. Grab the handles in such a way that you are using

27

your core to pull and push the handles in and out. To do this, you'll have to hold the handles at the lower parts or the midsection. Try as much as possible to have your arms positioned where your obliques are. It may seem strange and difficult at first, but practice makes perfect and you will get the hang of it eventually. When you have gotten the hang of it, then you may want to start using interval training along with strengthening your core to get max results. You can do the exercises listed above, but ensure your arms and body are positioned in the right way to get your abs working. Not only will your abs be put to the test, but so will your rear, because, as I mentioned before, your butt and ab muscles keep you upright and balanced.

You can also work your abs out by isolating your abs even more. You can do this by not using the handles at all. This is a very advanced move, so don't even bother trying unless you have the experience and the know-how to do this. You won't be going hands-free for the whole workout though, as you will be alternating between using your arms and not using them. When you start to get used to this workout and find that it is getting a bit easy, adjust the incline. Again, be very careful in this workout as you can seriously injure yourself.

Chapter 7: Building a Stronger Back

Earlier I mentioned a workout that involves the use of your back. In that workout, the back is brought in just by the positioning of the hands on the moving handles. The elliptical is a perfect machine for people with back and spinal problems, as it doesn't involve impact like the treadmill. On the treadmill, the user's foot hits the ground, but it is not so on the elliptical, where the foot is not even lifted and hardly moves around the knees. The machine also forces you to keep your back straight, and is the machine of choice for those with multiple sclerosis.

As mentioned before, to get the use of the lower back involved, you have to grab the middle or the lower parts of the handles. They should be positioned in such a way that when you are moving, it is as though you are rowing with your arms. To get the middle of your back, you just raise your arms so your hands are near the top of the handles. Here, you will bend your arms slightly. Do not use your arms to push and pull, but your back. This means that you should feel your shoulder blades going back and forth with each pedal. Then, to work your upper back, place your hands on top of the handles. Keep your arms straight, as this isolates your back muscles and lets them do the work instead of your arm muscles. In other words, your back will be doing the pushing and pulling.

Chapter 8: How to Tone the Arms

Not all elliptical machines come with the moving arm handles, but if you step on one that does, you will get a better body workout than on any other cardio machine. Even though most people use their arms less when doing this machine, the elliptical works out the arms as well as the legs. Apart from boxing, you will never get your arms to do any other more intense cardio exercise than what you can do with the elliptical machine.

If you want more toned arms, you will need to rely less on your legs and more on your arms. This is a hard thing, as your legs are the driving force in the elliptical, but sharing the load between your arms and legs will get you better all-round results.

To do this, don't hold the handles like you did before. Hold the bars either near the top of the handles or the very top. This time though, you will not be keeping your arms straight, but you will be bending and stretching your arm with each pedal. If you have your hand on the very top of the handles, position your elbows so it is pointing out to the sides, and bring the handle in in such a way that your arm is bent into a wing shape, then push it out again. You'll aid each arm with the other arm, so when one arm pulls, the other arm pushes. When you get your arms to cooperate like this, then you will take much of the work from your legs and you will give your arms the workout that they need. If you've skied before, then it will be a familiar movement.

Chapter 9: Toning Your Lower Half (Butt and Legs)

Get a Better Butt

If you ask any woman what part of the body she works out the most on the elliptical, then she will tell you it is her butt. The elliptical and the Stairmaster are the two best machines to get firmer and more toned glutes. Just as with any other workout done on the elliptical, working your glutes depends on how you position yourself and your range of motion.

To get a nicer butt you will need to both build muscle and also burn the fat underneath. Hence, you will be doing pretty much the same exercises in the same amount of time that you have done before, but you will be in different positions. To target your glutes, start off by warming up for about five minutes. Then, increase your resistance and ramp. Instead of pressing through the balls of your feet, use your heels instead. Do this for half of the workout time, then in the second half, switch to pedaling backwards.

The best thing to do in these workouts is to randomize your intensity levels. Most, if not all, elliptical machines will have a mode in which the user can choose how they want to use the machine. The random mode will alternate between high and low levels of resistance and ramp to help you get a better workout without having to take interval rests and cool down times. The random mode will do all this for you. So, when working out a single part of the body, especially your glutes, aim for the random mode as you will get a much better workout this way. Workouts should last between 15 and 30 minutes, followed by a 5 minute cool-down period.

Get Better Legs

Your legs are the parts of your body that get the most workout when on the elliptical machine. Even though your arms help out some or most of the time, it is your legs that move the platforms of the machine to keep them going. You'll find that it is very hard to move the elliptical machine with just your arms alone. The elliptical combines a range of motion that works your quads, hamstrings, calves and glutes. You can give your legs a better workout by using less of your arms with your workouts. You can do that by holding onto the stationary handles rather than the moving ones.

When using the elliptical, ensure that you position your feet well on the platform, and that your feet are shoulder-width apart. You can do exercises such as The Hill workout and The Ladder workout as detailed in the earlier chapters, but instead of placing your arms on the moving handles, keep them on the stationary handles instead. You can also do a simple workout where you go at a steady pace. You are more likely to burn fat while building muscle through HIIT workouts. If you do this in a forward motion, then you will be hitting your quads more. However, once you pedal backward, you will be hitting your hamstrings, calves and glutes.

You should also practice pedaling backwards without the use of your arms, or by taking your hands off the machine altogether. Doing this will isolate your inner thighs as well as your quads, butt and hamstrings in order to keep you balanced. Doing it this way will also increase calorie-burn, but this workout is for advanced users only. Stick to the basics until you are ready to go hands-free. To get better results, ensure that the ramp is at a medium to high range.

Conclusion

To get to your maximum cardiovascular potential and to lose the max amount of weight, do the exercises in this book at least three times a week. Remember you don't need more than 30 minutes, as it is all about the intensity of the workout. One important thing that wasn't mentioned in any of the chapters earlier is **stretching**. It is important to stretch after each session. Not only will you prevent injury, but you will also ensure proper blood flow to and away from your muscles and different areas of your body. Once blood is flowing, oxygen will flow faster, which will encourage more calories to be burned.

Sprinting is not a very comfortable exercise for many people, neither is cycling. The elliptical gives the butt-kicking intensity of HIIT cardio with comfort. It does feel weird at first, but in a few minutes, you will get the hang of it. If you want to get the maximum results, skip the treadmill and do 20 to 30 minutes on the elliptical instead. Your body will thank you for it. Top personal trainers will tell you that the elliptical is a powerhouse among cardio equipment, as it builds muscle strength and endurance in vital muscle groups, such as your quads, calves, back, arms and even your chest.

The purpose of this book is to give you options in using the elliptical machine. Don't just pick your favorite workout and then stick with that. It pays off to vary your workouts, as your muscles can get accustomed to your motion, and eventually burn less calories. Keep on surprising your body with the different cardio workouts provided here, and you will look great in no time!

Finally, I'd like to thank you for purchasing this book! If you found it helpful, I'd greatly appreciate it if you'd take a moment to leave a review on Amazon. Thank you!

Printed in Great Britain
by Amazon

49855817R00030